Weight
Nutrition
Guide

Weight Nutrition Guide

JORDAN YOUNG

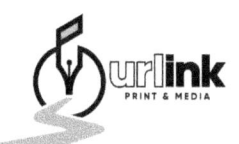

Weight Nutrition Guide

Copyright © 2019 by Jordan Young. All rights reserved.

No part of this publication may be reproduced, stored in a retrieval system or transmitted in any way by any means, electronic, mechanical, photocopy, recording or otherwise without the prior permission of the author except as provided by USA copyright law.

The opinions expressed by the author are not necessarily those of URLink Print and Media.

1603 Capitol Ave., Suite 310 Cheyenne, Wyoming USA 82001
1-888-980-6523 | admin@urlinkpublishing.com

URLink Print and Media is committed to excellence in the publishing industry.

Book design copyright © 2019 by URLink Print and Media. All rights reserved.

Published in the United States of America

ISBN 978-1-64367-959-4 (Paperback)
ISBN 978-1-64367-958-7 (Digital)

Non-Fiction
24.05.19

Contents

1. Healthful Ways Of Losing Weight 7
2. Healthful Steps In Losing Weight 9
3. Healthful Facts... 11
4. Low Calorie Foods That Are High In Nutrition 14
5. Essential Vitamins and Minerals for Good Health.. 15
6. Essential Nutritional Terms For Good Health.... 23
7. Foods To Keep Away From Or Restrict 26
8. Foods You Can Eat 29
9. All About Fiber 33
10. Water 35
11. The Meat and High-Protein Food Group 37
12. Sugar.. 39
13. Salt 41
14. Cholesterol... 43
15. An Exercise Program 46

Healthful Ways Of Losing Weight

If you are overweight and have been unsuccessful with countless diets and plans in the past, the following may be your answer to success. A thinner you will feel and look better. Some doctors believe that overweight is America's No.1 health problem and the cause of some heart disease. The following suggestions will help you control food intake and make the dieting experience more comfortable, while supplying your body with important nutrients. You must decide to eat less food and maintain a balance nutritional program.

However, before taking any weight control program, you need to convince yourself that you really want to feel better, look better and enjoy better health. Once you have decided the rest is quite straightforward. Also, once you start in a healthful nutritional program in losing pounds and inches, you may notice an improvement in your overall health. The idea is to make small, not drastic, changes in your otherwise normal everyday life.

Your diet should consist of both natural foods and vitamins. Try not to get all your vitamins from food alone. One of the advantages of eating natural foods and having a multiple vitamin is that they consist of all the enzymes, and minerals, and other substances necessary for the body to metabolize them. Also, eating a variety of natural foods and taking a multiple vitamin helps you to get your share of any vitamins or nutrients that have not yet been known.

Healthful Steps In Losing Weight

1. Try to always weigh yourself before breakfast, because this is the best time.
2. For a high energy drink, blend one banana with milk. You may add some wheat germ to this.
3. Try not to use drinks with caffeine in it. Drink postum or herb teas instead. Try herb tea with lemon.
4. Try to take a multiple vitamin supplement every day after meals. This will aid in maintaining daily requirements of essential nutrients.
5. Try not to eat more calories than your own body requires.
6. Try to do some form of exercise, like walking, bicycling or swimming. This will help burn off more calories and will develop muscle tone as well.
7. Try to eliminate all fats from your diet and most processed foods. Excess fats could overload the body chemistry.
8. Eat mainly fresh fruits, vegetables and whole-grain breads.
9. Before starting any diet, always check with your physician.
10. Try to avoid cake, pie, ice cream, doughnuts, chocolates, and rich desserts.

11. Reduce weight by eating <u>less</u> <u>calories</u>. Too much <u>sugar</u> and food containing <u>sugar</u> leads to overweight. Natural <u>fresh</u> <u>fruit</u> and <u>vegetables</u> are better for you.
12. Substitute lemon juice or vinegar in place of salad dressing made with oil or mayonnaise.
13. One particular food that is very effective in helping anyone lose weight is soup. Those who have soup for lunch generally consume fewer calories than those who do not have soup. Since soup is generally a water-based liquid, it usually has a lower caloric density than solid foods. The <u>broth</u> or <u>tomato</u> <u>based</u> <u>soups</u> have less calories and are the best choices.

The worse choice are the cream or oil-based soups which contain too much fat and too many calories. Try minestrone or vegetable soup with rice, barley, split peas, lentils, or rice.

When buying soups, buy the low sodium canned soups and no added fat contents. Flavor can be added to the soup by using salt free onion powder or salt free garlic powder.

Healthful Facts

1. Carbohydrates form the chief part of the diet in most parts of the world and hence are the major source of energy for most of the world's population. With the exception of meats, fats, salad oils, and a few other nutrients, almost everything we ingest contains carbohydrates.
2. Honey or artificial sweetener may be used in place of sugar.
3. Alcoholic beverages contain a lot of calories. Limiting your alcoholic intake to a glass of dry white wine per week or in very moderate quantity appears to be all right.
4. Sliced carrots (stored in water in the refrigerator) will provide a tasty crunchy snack when necessary.
5. It is healthier to eat whole wheat bread because it contains more nutrients. (Avoid white bread since when the flour is processed it loses essential nutrients. You want the most nutrition from whatever bulk food you do eat.)
6. The secret of cooking frozen vegetables successfully is to cook the vegetable until just tender. In this way you retain vitamins, bright color and fresh flavor. Frozen vegetables may be cooked in a small amount of water, steamed, or baked. Or they may be cooked in a covered fry pan.

7. There are no known advantages to consuming excess amounts of any nutrient.
8. To assure an adequate diet, a variety of foods should be eaten.
9. Fruit will improve a person's overall health, and satisfy your needs for sweets without refined sugar.
10. Fruit also adds fiber to your diet.
11. Pears, Peaches, Bananas, Apples and Oranges are excellent fruit for carbohydrates and nutrients.
12. Don't rely on weight as a measure of nutrition, for it is possible to be overweight and undernourished.
13. The best substitute for sugar is fruit and fruit juices.
14. Water has been called "the most essential nutrient." A person can live for weeks without food, but only for a few days without water.
15. A recommended cholesterol level is 160 milligrams per deciliter of blood, or 100 plus your age, whichever is lower. A desirable level of total blood cholesterol is less than 200 milligrams per deciliter (200mg/dl).
16. Hot Cereals like Barley and Oats may lower cholesterol.
17. By eating spicy foods, such as the condiment, horseradish, or the vegetable, chili peppers one might burn calories by causing a temporary rise in metabolic rate.
18. All vegetables are low in calories. Broccoli, asparagus, beets, carrots, celery, cucumbers, onions, peppers, tomatoes, lettuce, peas, corn, baked potato etc., and all are rich in vitamins and minerals.

19. Researchers believe a high-fiber diet keeps blood sugar levels in balance and may therefore help control diabetes. Some types of fiber-those found in fruits, legumes, vegetables, barley, oats, and brown rice-actually lower cholesterol.
20. A very nourishing drink is carrot juice. Fresh carrot juice contains all known minerals for the body. Raw carrot juice is rich in potassium, creates an alkaline balance, and works on the entire endocrine glandular system to issue valuable hormones needed by your scalp. Carrot juice also builds a nourishing bloodstream and strengthens the nervous system. Carrot juice can be mixed with raw celery and cucumber juice for added power.
21. Make your own fruit juice sparkler drink by mixing 1 part fruit juice and 2 parts plain seltzer.

Low Calorie Foods That Are High In Nutrition

Cauliflower	Turnips	Blueberries
Broccoli	Oranges	Blackstrap Molasses
Bell Peppers	Strawberries	Beets
Carrots	Iceberg Lettuce	Skim or non-fat milk
Spinach	Fresh Green Beans	Fresh Peaches
Tomatoes	Watermelon	Peaches canned in Light-syrup
Cantaloupe	Cucumbers	Low Fat Yoghurt
Radishes	Green Onions	Cream Style Corn
Romaine Lettuce	Snow Peas	Prune Juice
Boston Lettuce	Tuna in water	
Asparagus	Raw Celery	

Controlling weight is more than counting calories. When reducing calories-do not cut out basic foods. Eat wisely while eating less.

Essential Vitamins and Minerals for Good Health

VITAMINS

Vitamin A (Retinol) Vitamin A itself is found only in animal foods; the best sources are liver and fish liver oils (cod or halibut). Butter, cheese, eggs, and milk are good sources.

Good sources of carotene—from which the body can make Vitamin A-are the green leafy vegetables, carrots, sweet potatoes, squash, tomatoes, and the yellow fruits.

Corn is the only common cereal which contains carotene.

When absent in sufficient amounts, "night blindness" and other eye disorders, dry and brittle hair and skin, and infections of the mucous membranes may occur.

Cooking destroys vitamin A: thus overcooking should be avoided.

It is essential for the development and health of eyes, skin, hair, teeth and gums.

Vitamin C (ascorbic acid) It is not stored in the body.

All fresh, growing foods contain Vitamin C. The richest sources are the citrus fruits, guavas, ripe bell peppers, and rose hips. Tomato juice, fresh strawberries, and cabbage are fair sources.

It is essential in forming "collagen"—the substance that holds the cells of your body together. Lack of C may cause bleeding, swollen joints, and other complications. C is easily destroyed by heat and air. It is also the only vitamin which is not stored in body tissues and therefore, the body's requirement is needed every day.

It also aids utilization of iron.

<u>Vitamin D</u> The "<u>sunshine</u>" vitamin, naturally occurring in fish liver oils, and needed to help build strong bones and teeth. Regulates absorption of calcium and phosphorus to promote normal growth of bones and teeth.

Fish-liver oils and milk fortified with Vitamin D are the richest sources.

<u>Vitamin E (Tocopherol)</u> Vitamin E is not yet fully understood but its sole and vital function seems to be to prevent destruction by oxygen of unsaturated fatty acids and other fatlike substances. These include Vitamin A, the essential fatty acids, and the hormones of the pituitary, adrenal, and sex glands. Also, it inhibits coagulation of blood by preventing blood clots.

Good food sources are wheat germ, whole grains, vegetables, and leafy vegetables.

Vitamin E requirements are increased by the intake of polyunsaturated fats, but these fats are also the best sources of Vitamin E.

<u>Folic Acid (Folacin)</u> It is necessary for the division of body cells and for the production of RNA and DNA, the substances which carry hereditary patterns. As a coenzyme it is required for the utilization of sugar and amino acids. Folic acid is stored primarily in the liver.

Good food sources are liver, kidney, green vegetables, and nuts.

<u>Thiamine (B1)</u> Essential for normal function of nerve tissues, circulatory system and muscles. Promotes normal appetite, digestion and assimilation of foods. Helps get energy from food by promoting proper metabolism of sugars.

Good food sources are whole grain products, liver, fish, poultry, meat, milk and peas.

<u>Riboflavin (B2)</u> It plays an important role in both protein and energy metabolism, and is required for tissue oxidation and respiration. In combination with Vitamin A it is important in promoting good vision and healthy skin.

Good food sources are liver, milk, whole grain products, green leafy vegetables, fish and eggs.

<u>Niacin</u> (<u>B3</u>) (<u>Nicotinic acid</u>) Functions as a coenzyme in the oxidation of carbohydrates and is important in tissue respiration. It is needed for proper brain functions, the nervous system, and for a healthy skin.

Good food sources are lean meats, liver, wheat germ, milk and milk products, rice bran, fish and eggs.

<u>Pyridoxine (B6)</u> Aids in red blood cell formation and function of nervous system. Helps maintain the balance of sodium and potassium which regulates body fluids and promotes the normal functioning of the nervous and musculoskeletal systems.

The best sources of vitamin B6 are meats and whole grains. Other good food sources are Brewer's yeast, Blackstrap molasses, Green leafy vegetables, Legumes, and Desiccated liver.

<u>Vitamin (B12) (Cyanocobalamin)</u> It is necessary for normal metabolism of nerve tissue and is involved in protein, fat, and carbohydrate metabolism. Good food sources are milk, and milk products, fish, eggs, cheese, seafood and kidney beans.

<u>Biotin</u> A water-soluble B-complex vitamin. As a coenzyme, it assists in the making of fatty acids, and in the oxidation of fatty acids and carbohydrates. Without Biotin the body's fat production is impaired.

Good food sources are Egg yolks, liver, whole grains, sardines and legumes.

<u>Pantothenic Acid</u> Works with enzymes to convert carbohydrates, fats and proteins to energy. Needed for utilization of other B vitamins. Also required for formation of certain hormones and nerve regulating substances. The more stress one is under, the greater appears to be the need for pantothenic acid.

Good food sources are Egg yolks, legumes, whole grains, wheat germ, salmon, liver and green leafy vegetables.

MINERALS

<u>Calcium</u> A metallic element present in most animal and vegetable matter, and the most abundant mineral in the human body. It is essential for healthy teeth, bones, muscles, nerves, heart function and for normal blood clotting.

The richest sources are milk and milk products such as yogurt, cheese, and cultured buttermilk. Other sources are green leafy vegetables, molasses, and oily fish.

<u>Phosphorus</u> A nonmetallic element present in the tissues of all animals and plants. In biological tissues it is present in the form of phosphate. In humans 80 per cent of it is present in the skeletal and teeth, about 10 per cent in the muscles, and 1 per cent in the nervous system. It is of vital importance in metabolism; acts as a hardening agent in the bones and teeth; and is necessary for the proper functioning of the muscles and nerves.

Good food sources are milk and milk products, meat, fish, poultry, eggs, and whole grain cereals.

<u>Iodine</u> A nonmetallic element essential for the formation of thyroxine and triiodothyronine, the hormones secreted by the thyroid gland. Since the thyroid gland controls the basal metabolism of the

body, an undersupply of the thyroid hormones leads to fatigue, slowed pulse, low blood pressure, and a tendency to gain weight even though the calorie intake is small.

Iodine is found in minute amounts in all parts of the body, but it is particularly concentrated in the thyroid gland. (The body of the average adult contains about 40 milligrams of iodine, half of which is present in the thyroid gland.)

Much of the iodine once present in rocks and soil has been washed into the ocean. Consequently the only reliable sources of iodine are seafood and iodized salt. Dairy products, eggs, and some vegetables may be good sources, but they are undependable since the amount of iodine they contain varies with the amount of iodine in the soil from which they grow or from which the food they eat grows.

Bananas are also a good source of Iodine.

IRON is a mineral concentrate in the blood which is present in every living cell. All iron exists in the body combined with protein.

The major function of iron is to combine with protein and copper in making hemoglobin, the coloring matter of red blood cells. Hemoglobin transports oxygen in the blood from the lungs to the tissues, which need oxygen to maintain the basic life functions. Thus iron builds up the quality of the blood and increases resistance to stress and disease.

Good food sources are liver, lean meat, fish, poultry, Blackstrap Mollasses, and green leafy vegetables.

MAGNESIUM Acts as a catalyst in the utilization of carbohydrates, fats, protein, calcium, phosphorus, and possibly potassium. Combines with calcium and phosphorus to form bone tissues.

Good food sources are seafood, whole grains, molasses and dark green vegetables.

Copper A metallic element essential for the formation of hemoglobin (which carries oxygen throughout the body in the red blood cells) and the production of ribonucleic acid (RNA, which is part of the nucleus of every cell).

Good food sources are raisins, mushrooms, chocolate, seafood, and legumes.

ZINC A metallic vital element in skeletal growth and development, and essential for repair of injured tissues. Needed for utilization of carbohydrates, production of male hormones and metabolism of proteins.

Good food sources are liver, beans, seafood, sunflower seeds and mushrooms.

Vitamins are divided into two categories:

1. Fat-soluble vitamins A, D, E, and K. They occur in food in solution with fats and are stored in the body to a greater degree than the water-soluble

vitamins. These vitamins are mainly stored in the liver.
2. <u>Water-soluble vitamins</u> are members of the B vitamin complex and Vitamin C. There is no specific storage site in the body for the water-soluble vitamins. They are dispersed in solution through the blood and tissues.

Essential Nutritional Terms For Good Health

CALORIES

A term that signifies the amount of chemical energy that may be released as heat when food is metabolized. Therefore foods that are high in energy value are high in calories, while foods that are low in energy value are low in calories. Fats yield approximately nine calories per gram, and carbohydrates and proteins yield approximately four calories per gram.

Intake of food is measured in calories because the number of calories ingested is directly related to the energy available to the body. If the energy expended is less than that available, the usual result is weight gain.

Energy

The ability to do work. The energy the body requires for its metabolic processes, the maintenance of body temperature, and muscular activity, comes from the oxidation of foods, specifically, carbohydrates, fats, and whatever proteins are available after tissue building needs are met. The energy expended by the body is measured in the number of calories used. Energy is stored in the body as fat.

Carbohydrates

Carbohydrates are the chief source of energy for all body functions and muscular exertion and are necessary to assist in the digestion and assimilation of other foods. Carbohydrates provide us with immediately available calories for energy by producing heat in the body when carbon in the system unites with oxygen in the bloodstream. Carbohydrates also help regulate protein and fat metabolism; fats require carbohydrates for their breakdown within the liver.

The principal carbohydrates present in foods are sugars, starches, and cellulose. Simple sugars, such as those in honey and fruits, are very easily digested. Double sugars, such as table sugar, require some digestive action, but they are not nearly as complex as starches, such as those found in whole grain.

PROTEIN

Next to water, protein is the most plentiful substance in the body. Protein is one of the most important elements for the maintenance of good health and vitality and is of primary importance in the growth and development of all body tissues. It is the major source of building material for muscles, blood, skin, hair, nails, and internal organs, including the heart and the brain.

Most meats and dairy products are complete-protein foods, while most vegetables and fruits are incomplete-protein foods.

Fats

Fats, or lipids, are the most concentrated source of energy in the diet. When oxidized, fats furnish more than twice the number of calories per gram furnished by carbohydrates or proteins. One gram of fat yields approximately nine calories to the body.

In addition to providing energy, fats act as carriers for the fat-soluble vitamins, A, D, E, and K.

Fat supplies essential fatty acids needed for growth, health, and smooth skin. Fats are either saturated or unsaturated. Natural vegetable oils are rich sources of unsaturated fats and are preferred to the saturated animal fats to reduce cholesterol levels.

Safflower oil contains the highest amount of the essential fatty acids and the greatest amount of linoleic acid, the most important of them.

Fatty meats, butter, cream, egg yolk, and lard are sources of saturated fats.

Foods To Keep Away From Or Restrict

SOURCES OF CHOLESTEROL IN OUR DIET

TOP FIVE FOODS	PERCENTAGE OF DIETARY CHOLESTEROL
EGGS _____	35.9%
BEEF STEAKS, ROASTS _____	8.7%
HAMBURGERS, MEAT LOAF __	7.3%
WHOLE MILK _____	5.4%
HOT DOGS, HAM, _____ LUNCH MEATS	4.3%

SOURCES OF FAT IN OUR DIET

TOP FIVE FOODS	PERCENTAGE OF DIETARY FAT
BURGERS, MEAT LOAF	7.02%
HOT DOGS, HAM, LUNCH MEATS	6.39%
WHOLE MILK, WHOLE MILK BEVERAGES	5.98%
DOUGHNUTS, CAKES, COOKIES	5.98%
BEEF STEAKS, ROASTS	5.45%

What is Cholesterol? Chemically it is a fatty alcohol naturally occurring in the bile used in the stomach. When produced in excess (by eating too much fat) it is believed to form a hard, insoluble deposit on the inner walls of the blood vessels. This narrows them down, raising their resistance to blood flow and hence building up blood pressure. Excess cholesterol is now called a major cause of hardening of the arteries-a major cause of death. The excess can be controlled by avoiding saturated fats and by drug therapy. The common dietary fats are essential to body metabolism, in moderation.

Cholesterol must not be thought of as being all villain. In addition to being an essential part of every living cell, it is the base molecule from which the sex hormones and the hormones of the adrenal gland are formed.

Fats

Saturated Fats, the Undesirable Fat: These fats come from meats and dairy products and are usually solid at room temperature. Saturated fats may cause our bodies to form cholesterol and raise the level of cholesterol in the blood. This relates to coronary heart disease.

Unsaturated Fats, the Desirable Fat: Are mostly liquid and include mainly the vegetable oils.

Polyunsaturated fats are usually liquid at room temperature and are found mainly in plants. Safflower oil, corn oil, and soybean oil are examples.

<u>Monounsaturated fats</u> such as Olive oil and Peanut Oil are also liquid at room temperature, but tend to become solid when placed in the refrigerator for a few days.

<u>Safflower oil</u> contains the highest amount of the essential fatty acids and the greatest amount of linoleic acid, the most important of them.

Foods You Can Eat

"<u>DAIRY</u> <u>PRODUCTS</u>" Reduce the amount of dairy products that you normally eat. Plain lowfat Yogurt
Skim milk (has the same Calcium value as whole milk and provides the same nutritional value as you get from regular milk)

Powdered skim milk, 1/3 cup
Nonfat dry milk (quantity needed to make one cup)
Low Fat Cottage Cheese, 1% FAT
Low Fat American Cheese

The nutrition program limits your dairy servings because even small helpings of dairy are <u>high</u> <u>in</u> <u>calories and fat</u>. You will find a number of varieties of low fat cottage cheeses and yogurt on supermarket shelves, and these along with low fat milk and low fat cheeses eaten from time to time, should be all the dairy foods you require.

"<u>Protein</u>" Should be about 15-20% of total calories.
A meat serving is usually a lean, cooked portion.
Chicken (white meat, no skin)
Dried peas, beans, ¼ cup cooked
Flounder

Haddock   Mackerel   Natural Peanut Butter, 2 teaspoons

Halibut	Navy beans	Salmon, 1 ounce
Lamb	Other legumes	Sardines, 1 ounce
Sprouts	Pinto beans	Sole, 2 ounces
Tongue	Red beans	Tuna (water-packed), 2 Ounces
	Soybeans	

It takes 2 ounces of fish (as opposed to 1 ounce of meat) to provide 50 calories. So eating fish enables you to have larger servings and still stay within your daily limit. You may want to increase your intake of this food item.

Excess Protein increases the risk of <u>osteoporosis</u> (weakening of the bones due to calcium loss)

Protein deficiency produces kwashiorkor. In this condition there may be pot belly, skin rash, and hair color changes; the hair frequently falls out.

"<u>Mineral</u> <u>Vegetables</u>"

Dark green leafy vegetables like spinach, kale, lettuce, and broccoli are high in minerals, such as <u>magnesium</u> and <u>potassium</u> (which effect blood-pressure regulation) and <u>calcium</u> (which helps to prevent osteoporosis).

Spinach	Fresh Cauliflower	Kelp
Sweet Potato	Chopped Cabbage	Okra
Potato	Fresh Artichoke	Radishes
Kale, Fresh	Fresh Green Beans	Scallions
Winter Squash	Summer Squash	Soups (noncreamed, vegetable only)

Fresh Broccoli	Turnips	
Fresh Asparagus	Bean Sprouts	Tomato sauce (⅓ cup)
Frozen mixed Vegetables		
Eggplant	All vegetable juices	
Tomatoes	Romaine Lettuce	Zucchini
Carrots	Chopped Onion	
Frozen Green Peas	Cucumber	
Green Pepper	Beets	
Fresh Sweet Corn	Celery	

"<u>Fruits</u>"

These are unrefined simple carbohydrates and will make up between 5 percent and 10 percent of your total carbohydrate food consumption. Eating fruit enables you to sharply reduce your intake of refined sugar. Fruits rank high on the list of whole foods. Eat the whole fruit in preference to drinking fruit juices whenever you can. Fruit will maintain your energy level and satisfy your hunger between meals.

Watermelon	Honeydew Melon	Blueberries
Papaya	Strawberries	Fresh Pineapple
Cantaloupe	Raspberries	Cherries
Mango	Peach	Pomegranate
Orange	Prunes	Red Plums
Grapefruit	Tangerine	Grapes
Banana	Apple	

"Grains and Carbohydrate Vegetables"

Grain Group: Whole or enriched grains, whole wheat bread in any shape, hot or cold cereals, macaroni, noodles, or other pasta. Neither pasta or potatoes are fattening. A large dish of pasta uses 2 of your daily grain and carbohydrate portions.

Barley	Dried peas or beans	Parsnips
Beans	English muffin	Pasta
Bran muffin	Garbanzo beans	Rice cakes
Brown rice	Green peas	Yams
Buckwheat	Hot cereal	Winter squash
Bulgur	Kasha	Whole wheat bread
Cold cereal	Soups (meatless, noncreamed bean)	
Corn bread	Whole grain bread	
Corn muffin	White potato	Soybean flour
Crackers, unsalted	Sweet potato	Rye flour
Oat meal	Spaghetti squash	Soybeans

> The First Wealth Is Health and
> There is nothing better Than A Healthy Diet.

Eat more fresh fruits, vegetables, and whole grain products while eating less meat and dairy products.

Watch out for the deadly five, fat, alcohol, cholesterol, salt, and sugar.

All About Fiber

Fiber or roughage is very important in the human diet. Fiber refers to the part of food that is not digested or absorbed by the human body, such as the skin of an apple.

Also, fiber helps speed the passage of food through the dietary tract. Much of this natural aid to proper digestion and elimination is missing from the foods many people eat. The normal functioning of the intestinal tract depends on the presence of adequate fiber. A low-fiber diet has been associated with heart disease, cancer of the colon and rectum, diverticulosis, varicose veins, phlebitis, and obesity.

Apples and bananas contain valuable bulk fiber in the form of indigestible cellulose, which is needed for regular bowel movement. Bananas are high in magnesium and may be useful for treatment of diarrhea, colitis, ulcers, and certain cases of protein allergies. Bananas and pears are the highest in natural sugars.

There are 2 types of fiber: soluble and insoluble. Both types are recommended as important parts of a healthful, well-balanced diet. Only soluble fiber has a cholesterol-lowering effect. Soluble fiber is found in foods such as fruits, vegetables, rolled oats, oat bran, barley and beans.

Whole wheat bread, fresh fruit and vegetables are an excellent source of fiber, and the dark green leafy vegetables have some of the highest amounts. Other good sources of fiber include whole grains, whole grain flours, whole baked potatoes with skin, high fiber and bran cereals, and beans.

Fiber keeps the entire gastro intestinal system functioning smoothly.

Water

Water is our most important nutrient. Water is a clear, colorless, nearly odorless and tasteless liquid without which most plant and animal life cannot live. Chemically a compound composed of hydrogen and oxygen (H_2O), it forms more than 60 per cent of the body weight of humans, and obviously plays an important role in metabolism. It has been demonstrated that the younger the animal, the richer it is in water; and the fatter the animal, the smaller is the percentage of water.

As a solvent water aids in the absorption of water-soluble nutrients and in the elimination of water soluble waste through the urine (and to some extent through the feces.) Also, by means of the evaporation of water through the skin in perspiration and by way of the lungs in exhalation, water plays an important role in the control of body temperature.

Water provides neither vitamins nor calories, but it does provide various minerals: magnesium and calcium in hard water, and fluoride in water that either naturally contains it or to which it has been added by man. In addition, some specific mineral and spring waters contain mineral salts (carbonates, silicates, and chlorides) and iron.

A moderately active person in good health takes in an average of 5.5 pints of water per day. Approximately

3 pints of this comes from water and beverages containing water (coffee, tea, soft drinks, etc.), and 2.5 pints from solid foods (vegetables, fruits, meat, etc.) and liquid foods (soup, milk, etc.) containing water.

About 60 per cent of this intake is eliminated through the urine, 25 per cent through the skin (perspiration), 12 per cent through the lungs (vapor in the air exhaled) and 3 per cent in the feces.

When there is an unusual loss of water from the body (excessive perspiration in hot weather or from undue physical activity), the water should be replaced. Also, since water contains salt, it, too, should be replaced.

A human being can live for weeks without food, but only a few days without water.

An increase in water intake can actually reduce fat deposits while a decrease in water intake will cause fat deposits to increase.

It is suggested that 6 to 8 glasses of water a day is considered healthy.

The Meat and High-Protein Food Group

This group includes meat, fish, poultry, eggs, and such alternate vegetable items as dried beans, peas, and nuts. In addition to their protein contribution, these foods are a major source of the B-group vitamins and iron. They are rich in readily absorbed iron themselves, and they increase the availability of the iron in any vegetable foods eaten with them.

All meats are good sources of protein and vitamins B1, B2, and niacin.

They are also good sources of iron and phosphate.

The most healthful and nutritious servings in this group should come from fish, chicken, turkey, water packed tuna, and high-protein vegetable alternates such as beans, peas, nuts, and tofu.

There are basically two types of protein, complete protein and incomplete protein.

The richest sources of protein are those containing the eight essential amino acids, the complete proteins, in the greatest amounts—are egg yolk, fresh milk, liver and kidney.

Muscle meats (roasts, steaks, and chops) seafood, and cheese provide complete protein but contain a smaller amount of some of the essential amino acids than those cited above. Protein from brewer's yeast, wheat germ, soybeans and certain nuts are also complete proteins.

Incomplete protein lacks certain essential amino acids and is not used efficiently when eaten alone. Peas, most kinds of beans, cereals, lentils (peas and seeds), nuts, grains, and processed flour provide incomplete protein.

In short, animal proteins (meat, fish, and dairy products) provide the essential amino acids in greater amounts than do vegetable proteins.

Mixing complete and incomplete proteins can give you better nutrition than either one alone. Remember meats represent the end of the food chain, and contains additives and preservatives as well as pesticides.

Sugar

A white, crystalline refined carbohydrate substance obtained mainly from two plants, sugar cane and sugar beet. The extraction and refining process for both is similar, and both in their refined states are pure sucrose, containing neither vitamins nor minerals.

Natural sugars, such as those occurring in fruits, grains, milk and honey, normally provide all the sugar the body requires for energy and the typical American overconsumption of refined sugar does not benefit health.

Also, an excessive indulgence in soft drinks, bakery goods, and candies increases the need for vitamins, and elevates the blood-sugar level-an elevation usually followed by a sudden drop to a low blood sugar level which can result in fatigue, blackouts and fainting. It also leads to a feeling of great hunger, ensuing overeating and unwanted weight gain.

The average American consumes 120 pounds of sugar a year. This can lead to problems of tooth decay, overweight and possible diabetes.

FOODS HIGH IN SUGAR

Tonic, soda
Cookies, cakes, pastries, doughnuts
All types of candy and breath mints

Jelly, jam, honey, syrup
Ice-cream, ice milk, frozen yogurt, popsicles
Sugar-coated cereals
thick shakes, frappes
Fruit canned in heavy syrup
Instant cocoa
Coffee or tea with 1 or more teaspoons of sugar

Salt

Salt is a white crystal known as sodium chloride. Salt can contribute to high blood pressure or hypertension. Restricting salt to your diet can keep you from being hypertensive. A salt-free diet is not 100% salt free, since foods in general contain salt even if no salt is added. Salt is one of the essentials without which we cannot live.

Salt tends to hold fluid in the tissues and to cause edema. The most natural diuretic is to cut down on salt intake. In the United States the typical diet has ten times the required amount of salt; many authorities feel that this is one cause of high blood pressure and arteriosclerosis. No matter how hard you try to eliminate salt from your diet, you will still have more than enough. If you can eliminate some salt, you may have less edema and fluid retention. If food tastes flat without salt, try using lemon juice as a substitute. The commercial salt substitutes are also satisfactory.

Products with the word "<u>sodium</u>" or the symbol "<u>Na</u>" anywhere in the list of ingredients contain salt.

<u>FOODS HIGH IN SALT OR SODIUM:</u>
Processed foods such as canned vegetables, soups, luncheon meats, TV dinners, and processed cheese.

Also, snack foods such as corn chips, potato chips, pretzels, and salted nuts.

A high sodium diet can lead to high blood pressure, which increases a person's chance of developing heart disease.

Cholesterol

Cholesterol is a lipid or fat-like substance found in all foods of animal origin. It is a normal component of most body tissues occurring especially in the brain, bile, blood cells, plasma, liver and kidney of humans and animals, and in milk products, egg yolk, and animal fats and oils.

Many researchers believe cholesterol to be an important factor in causing various cardiovascular diseases. A diet rich in the saturated fatty acids (found chiefly in meats and dairy products) causes a rise in the blood cholesterol. Conversely, if the diet contains mostly unsaturated fatty acids (from vegetables and fish) the blood cholesterol will usually be lowered.

Cholesterol is not all bad. Our bodies use it to build cell membranes and produce important hormones. Even if you are on a cholesterol free diet, your liver manufactures cholesterol to keep your body supplied. Also, cholesterol is manufactured from starch and sugar by the liver whether or not cholesterol has been excluded from the diet.

There are two types of cholesterol. The bad cholesterol is known as low density lipoprotein (LDL). The good cholesterol is high density lipoprotein (HDL).

Bad cholesterol can be lowered by avoiding foods containing large amounts of cholesterol and certain fats called saturated fats. Saturated fats are found primarily in foods of animal origin, such as butter, cheese, and meat.

Good cholesterol contains the greatest amount of protein and the smallest amount of cholesterol.

Good cholesterol levels can be increased by exercising vigorously, not smoking, and losing weight if necessary.

A diet that will help you decrease your bad cholesterol and help control your cholesterol level is as follows.

1. Choose fish, poultry, lean meats, or beans for entrees.
2. Choose low-fat or better yet non-fat dairy products.
3. Eat more vegetables and fruits.
4. Eat a diet high in fiber.

Remember to drink more fluids as you take in more fiber. Fluids help the fiber move through your system.

5. Avoid commercially prepared baked products.
6. Broil, bake, or boil rather than fry.
7. Read labels to determine both amount and types of fat contained in foods.

Some foods, such as vegetables, fruits, cereals, grains and nuts, do not contain any cholesterol.

Eating the proper foods, along with moderate exercise and losing weight if necessary, can make a difference in your blood cholesterol level. Saturated fat in our diets is the main culprit in raising blood cholesterol.

An Exercise Program

Exercise should be part of everyone's nutritional program. Before beginning any type of exercise, you should consult with a physician to avoid any injury to your health, and to be sure there are no restrictions.

The key to any type of exercise is trying to motivate oneself to improve one's physical condition.

No matter what type of exercise you get involved in, whether you walk, go swimming, jog, play basketball, run, go skiing, go bicycling (regular or stationary) and so on, you should begin slowly and use common sense. The benefits of exercising are infinite. Regular physical exercise is both a good way to restore optimal health, reduce weight, decrease sodium, strengthen the cardiovascular system, reduce the risk of heart disease, decrease your blood sugar and blood fats, reduce fatigue and raise energy levels, counter the aging process, strengthen your muscles, relieve nervous tension, depression and anxiety, and gives you more vigor and vitality. It can also help control diabetes, which is another risk factor for heart disease.

Most experts recommend aerobic exercise such as cycling or jogging. To maintain aerobic fitness, the frequency and duration of exercise is important. Frequency should be three to four times per week, for a duration of 20 to 30 minutes.

www.ingramcontent.com/pod-product-compliance
Lightning Source LLC
LaVergne TN
LVHW021741060526
838200LV00052B/3400